ABNORMAL PSYCHOLOGY:

THE CAUSES AND TREATMENTS OF DEPRESSION, ANXIETY AND MORE
THIRD EDITION

CONNOR WHITELEY

ACKNOWLEDGMENTS
Thank you to all my readers without you I couldn't do what I love.

INTRODUCTION

If you've read any of my other books, then you know that I hate long boring introductions so I'll make this one short and filled with great interesting information for you.

<u>A Quick Note on Abnormal Psychology:</u>

Abnormal psychology is the study of patterns of behaviour that deviate from the accepted norms of society, but abnormal psychology doesn't study all deviations. Only those that can be classed as mental disorders.

Therefore, in this book, we will look at the causes of Major Depression Disorder (MDD) amongst other conditions and how disorders are diagnosed.

<u>So Who Am I?</u>

I'm Connor Whiteley and I'm a university

psychology student studying Psychology with Clinical Psychology with a year of work experience at the University of Kent in the United Kingdom.

And I LOVE mental conditions, abnormal psychology and clinical psychology.

Also, I'm the author of over 20 books and 11 of these books are psychology books.

Personally, I hate the term mental disorder or illness so you will very rarely see that term being used in this book and in my Clinical Psychology book I explain why I hate those terms in a lot more depth.

Who Is This Book For?

Well, that is a significant question and this book is for anyone interested in psychology, depression, mental conditions and treatment.

As in the book, I go into depression and other conditions as well as the wide range of treatment for these disorders.

Note: I hate long, boring complex books myself so please except this book to be easy to understand, engaging and filled with great information in short chapters!

Why Talk About Mental Conditions?

Personally, the reason why I write these books,

and I actively talk about mental health difficulties and conditions in my books and on The Psychology World Podcast, is because mental health is still stigmatised. Also, there is so many stereotypes and damaging opinions about mental health.

Therefore, if I can make any difference to change this and help people then I want to take that chance.

For example, I doubt any lay people are reading this book. (Yes, I hate the term lay people and yes, I think it's offensive) But people, in general, have a terrible understanding of mental health conditions.

Such as, people tend to think murders all have mental health conditions. Like: schizophrenia or they're psychopaths.

In reality, 95% of murderers have no mental health conditions.

In addition, 35% of people believe people who have a mental health condition are violent.

The reality is it is the small percentage of these people who are violent, and I talk more about this in my Forensic Psychology book, but the only reason why there's a higher rate of criminality in the mentally 'ill' population is because it's a smaller population as a whole.

So now that the introduction is done, please join

me on this journey of discovery as we explore the amazing topic of abnormal psychology.

But first, we need to look at what is Depression?

CHAPTER 1: WHAT IS DEPRESSION?
What Is Major Depression Disorder?

Let's face it feeling depressed is normal and a part of life. When you experience a break up or something bad happens to you. Then you'll likely feel depressed.

I know this from personal experience.

However, Major Depression Disorder (I prefer the term condition) is when you feel depressed for a long period of time.

When you get further into the book, I'll explain what the Diagnostic and Statistical Manual 5 is, but according to this manual depression is feeling sad and helpless for over two weeks. Also, it includes several symptoms. Including:

- Little energy

- Feelings of worthlessness and hopelessness
- Difficulty sleeping and concentration
- Suicidal thoughts
- Anhedonia

The last point is the inability to feel pleasure in an activity you normally get pleasure from. For example, if you love gardening or watching TV. You probably wouldn't be able to get pleasure from these activities if you had depression.

Personally, I would know something is seriously wrong if I no longer enjoyed psychology, and chances are you would too.

Statistics on Major Depression Disorder (Condition)
On a quick side note, I want to mention that depression is a common mental health condition because the lifetime prevalence of depression is 15%

Meaning over the course of your lifetime, there's a 15% chance you will get depression with the average age of onset being 27 years old.

Although unlike many of the mental health conditions, we look at in this book, Major Depression Disorder has an equal gender ratio.

In other words, it affects both genders equally and for every man who has depression. There is a woman who has depression as well.

What's the Difference Between Depression And

Bipolar Disorder?

I thought that I'll quickly mention this as I and a lot of friends didn't know the difference between these two conditions until another one of my friends had bipolar.

Therefore, unlike depression, people with bipolar disorder suffer maniac; extreme happiness; and depressive episodes that can last for hours, days or even weeks. In between these episodes, the person's mood is 'normal'

Interestingly, mania and depressive episodes can occur at the same time as people experience both tearfulness with grandiosity as well as menacing thoughts.

Although, in a milder maniac episode hypomania can occur. This is where the sufferer seems extremely talkative, tireless, infectiously merry and charming.

However, I know that the idea of hypomania sounds great as who doesn't want to be extremely happy. There are of course downsides.

For example, despite hypomanic feelings, it can cause a person to become overconfident and relentlessly pursue goals. (Johnsons, 2005)

This leads to a lot of other problems for the sufferer.

On the other hand as a final interesting fact, a person's metabolization (using/ breakdown) of glucose (sugar) increases during periods of mania and decreases during periods of depression.

What is Seasonal Affective Disorder?

Moving onto our final type of depression, I want to quickly look at Seasonal Affective Disorder because I read about the condition a few years ago in a textbook, and I was interested. I thought it was interesting that the change of season could impact a person's mood so severely.

Then it was a couple of years later when I learned about embodied social cognition and other cognitive processes that made the weather impacting our mood make sense to me.

Anyway, Seasonal Affective Disorder or SAD is a form of depression that regularly occurs during a particular season. Like winter. As well as clients with SAD have phase-delayed sleep and temperature rhythms, most depressed people have phase advanced patterns.

In short, their body clock is longer than the average person's and I discuss this topic a lot more in Biological Psychology.

To treat SAD, very bright lights can be used, and this is thought to work because the light affects the serotonin synapses and alters the circadian rhythm to help the client sleep better.

PART ONE: HISTORY AND DIAGNOSIS

CHAPTER 2: INTRODUCTION TO THE HISTORY OF MENTAL HEALTH

Before we dive into the actual content of the book, I think it's important to note how far we've come in terms of our thinking on mental disorders.

Now, I've used the term 'mental disorders' in this chapter because I want to highlight the fact that we used to and to some extent still do see mental conditions in an extremely negative light.

For example, autism is classed as a mental disorder but I've met tens of autistic people who were on various points on the spectrum, and they all said that autism is a gift and not a mental disorder.

Another favourite example of mine is a TED talk that I was shown in 6th Form or High School and it was a schizophrenic woman who was talking about her condition. It only became a problem for her when society told her that she had a problem and that she was abnormal.

Hence, showing you the damage that language and terminology can have on a person.

It's just something to think about.

The History of Mental Disorders:

Below is a quick whirlwind tour of the historical beliefs surrounding mental conditions.

Demonology:

Firstly, it was believed that mental conditions were caused by demonic possession and the beliefs surrounding mental health were tied into religious or spiritual beliefs.

Resulting in the treatment being about expelling the demon from the body.

Somatogenic:

After science had progressed a little, we thought; and this is partially true; that mental illnesses were caused by bodily or physical illnesses.

This is a good start as the body can play a role in the development of a condition, but there are other factors involved. Like: social and cognitive factors.

These will be spoken about in more depth later in the book.

One example of this hypothesis or way of thinking during the 1800s was General Paresis as it is caused by an infection of syphilis- with the following bodily symptoms:

- Fatigue
- Dizziness
- Personality changes and cognitive deterioration
- Delusion
- Subtle motor symptoms
- Death
- Dementia
- Catatonic

Somatogenic Hypothesis:

As a result of General Paresis being a severe problem, Orchard Von Kraft-Ebling (1897) used the somatogenic hypothesis to propose that paresis is caused by a syphilis infection.

Overall, the hypothesis proposes that mental illnesses come from physical illnesses or infections.

Classification:

Moving onto something that is still widely used in modern practice is the classification systems and there is a whole chapter dedicated to these interesting systems and diagnosis in the next chapter.

However, it all began with Emil Kraeplin (1856-1926) and he stated that mental illnesses come from a problem our brain biology.

In addition, he created a new classification system that grouped clusters of symptoms together or patterns instead of groups of similar symptoms.

The first categories that he formed were manic depression; now know as bipolar and major depression; and dementia praecox. Now known as schizophrenia.

So, his work was important as it gave us a foundation for the classification systems of modern practice and it's hard to deny that whilst the classification systems aren't perfect. They are useful.

However, I'm not a big fan of him as he was controversial as he wrote on 'radical hygiene' and eugenics.

Psychogenesis:

Now we're starting to move into more modern ways of thinking as psychogenesis appreciates that not everything is down to our biology and that there are psychological causes to mental conditions.

A great and classic example of psychogenesis is, hysteria as it was described by Freud as partially paralysing young women but there were no physical symptoms and the symptoms disappeared under hypnosis.

Leading Freud to develop this famous theory.

Note: while the Iceberg theory isn't correct, it was very important to introduce the idea of the unconscious and this theory has had a massive impact on modern theories.

For more information on Consciousness, please check out Cognitive Psychology.

PSYCHOGENIC HYPOTHESIS:

Iceberg Theory:

So Freud believed that unconscious psychological processes are in constant conflict.

Meaning in terms of mental illness, his hypothesis proposes that mental illness results as your defensive thoughts or behaviours try to reduce this internal conflict.

Just to reiterate, Freud is often unfairly rejected immediately but he has been very influential, and his findings have provided us with a foundation for a lot of areas. For example:

- Childhood development
- How trauma influences later life
- Sexuality

- Talking therapy
- Mediation

To summarise, the psychogenesis approach believes that mental illnesses have psychological causes, as well as Freud, believed that mental illnesses were caused by your defensive behaviours or thoughts trying to reduce this internal conflict.

Modern Approaches:

Moving onto one of my favourite areas, which are the more interesting models that we use in modern times. Including, my absolute favourite model called the biopsychosocial model.

We'll now look at what modern psychology thinks causes mental conditions to develop.

Diathesis-Stress Model:

This model proposes that mental illness manifests only if you are genetically deposited to the condition and there's a lot of stress that causes the condition to manifest, as well as this explains differences in reactions to stressors.

For example, if you're genetically deposited to develop depression and your parent or carer sadly dies. This causes you stress. Leading to the stress and genetics interacting. Resulting in the increased likelihood of you developing depression.

Overall, I want to stress that genetic factors can increase the risk of developing a mental condition, but it does NOT cause the condition itself.

Later in the book, I'll explain how different biological, psychological and social factors can cause depression and other conditions.

Another modern model is the biopsychosocial model; first proposed by George Engel in 1977; and this model looks at the interaction of biological, psychological and social factors to cause a physical and psychological condition to develop.

Hopefully, you've enjoyed this brief summary to the History of Mental Disorders and now we're going to look at diagnosis.

How does a sufferer of a mental condition get the diagnosis and the help they need?

CHAPTER 3: DIAGNOSIS

I will be the first to admit that there will be tons of information that I could include in this section and I could easily write three chapters on the topic of diagnosis and go into great depth.

However, this could make this book that is meant to be an introduction more of a long, boring book filled with dry information.

Basically, you'll put the book down in seconds.

Nevertheless, I'll compress the needed information into interesting manageable chunks.

Firstly, we'll look at what is abnormality?

Think about it, what does abnormality mean to you?

There are several theories that we'll look at now.

Abnormality as A Deviation from Social Norms:

This theory states the abnormality is something that isn't 'acceptable' in society.

While this is a good common-sense approach and the approach that I personally use, but a limitation of this theory is that social norms change over time.

For example, homosexuality was classified as a mental disorder and wasn't classed as a social norm until it was legalised in the UK in 1967. Only then could this behaviour be classed as normal.

Abnormality as Inadequate Functioning:

This theory belongs to Rosenhan and Seligman (1989) and it proposes 7 criteria that can be used to define abnormality.

Those 7 are:

- Suffering
- Maladaptive (for instance: not being able to achieve life goals)
- Unconventional behaviour (behaviour than not a lot of people do)
- Unpredictable behaviour
- Being irrational (so you can't understand why they behave that way)

- Observer discomfort (it makes you uncomfortable to watch the behaviour)
- Violation of moral standards

A strength is that the theory embraces more dimensions of what abnormality is. Such as socially unacceptable behaviour causes suffering to the person.

A weakness is that very few disorders meet all 7 criteria, so are they not abnormal behaviour?

<u>Abnormality as a deviation from ideal mental health:</u>

This theory was proposed by Jahoda (1958) and for her theory, she used the idea of ideal health. Therefore, she thought that it was more important to define what health is than abnormal behaviour.

She proposed the following as indicators of ideal mental health:

- Voluntary control of behaviour
- You have to have positive relationships
- You need to be productive.
- You need to have an accurate perception of the world.
- You need to have efficient self-perception.
- You need to have realistic self-esteem.

A strength is that the theory is more humanistic as it focuses on health over disorders.

Although, as not many people would meet all six, then is everyone not entirely healthy?

Modern Definitions:

However, there are currently two widely used modern definitions of abnormality and what a mental condition actually is.

"Mental, behavioural and neurodevelopmental disorders are syndromes characterized by clinically significant disturbance in an individual's cognition, emotional regulation, or behaviour that reflects a dysfunction in the psychological, biological, or developmental processes that underlie mental and behavioural functioning. These disturbances are usually associated with distress or impairment in personal, family, social, educational, occupational, or other important areas of functioning." (WHO, 2018).

In other words, the World Health Organisation defines mental disorders as syndromes that cause significant disturbances in a person's mental processes, emotions and behaviours that are caused by a wide range of factors.

Whereas the American Psychological Association defines mental disorders as:

"A mental disorder is a behavioural or psychological syndrome characterized by clinically significant disturbance or disability in an individual's cognition, emotion regulation, or behavior. Mental disorders are usually associated with significant distress or disability in social, occupational, or other important activities." (APA, 2013).

As briefly touched upon by the definitions, there's a wide range of factors that can cause a mental condition to develop. Including: biological, psychological and social factors.

Note: we will explore how each of these types of factors impacts depression later in the book.

Examples of Biological factors include:

- Gender
- Physical illnesses
- Disability
- Genetic predisposition
- Neurochemistry- these include deficits in certain neurotransmitters.
- Physiological response
- Stress reactivity
- Medication effects

Some examples of psychological or cognitive factors include:

- Emotions
- Thinking
- Perceptions

- Impact of past trauma
- Attitudes
- Values
- Self-esteem
- Coping and social skills
- Personality

Examples of social factors include:

- Religion
- Poverty
- Peer group
- Physical exercise
- Interpersonal relationships- like the relationship you have with your family and friends.
- Education
- Culture
- Family background
- Social support
- Medical care

Other Causes of Mental Disorders:

To wrap up this section on what causes conditions, I want to highlight:

- The Psychodynamic Approach- Freud believed disorders originated because of conflicts between the Id, ego and superego.

I know, I know why am I talking about Freud. But I mention to highlight this is an interesting idea that is ultimately wrong. Yet it provided a basis for modern ideas about psychological causes to grow.

- Medical- Hippocrates believed mental conditions originated from biological abnormalities.

If you ever read my <u>Clinical Psychology</u> book, you'll know how far back clinical psychology goes, but I want to mention how long people have been interested in learning about mental conditions.

This is something we'll look at throughout the book.

- The Cognitive Approach- mental conditions are caused by mental or psychological processes.

Personally, I love this approach to behaviour as I think this is really interesting.

Again, this is a common theme you'll see throughout the book when we get into the causes of the different conditions.

<u>Classification Systems:</u>

A classification system is a diagnostic manual providing a set of symptoms, a system of diagnostic categories (the type of disorder) as well as rules for making a diagnosis on these set of symptoms.

China uses its own manual called: the Chinese Classification of Mental Disorders (CCMD-3) and it's widely used by some other countries as well.

The World Health Organisation uses the International Classification of Diseases (ICD-10) and it's used in many European countries. Before an edition is published it has to be approved by all WHO members.

Building upon this further, the ICD-10 covers all aspects of health but chapter 5 covers 'Mental and Behavioural Disorders' using the code F00-F99

These codes are due to change in the ICD-11.

Therefore, these codes are as followed:

<u>F00-F09 Are Organic Including Symptoms of Symptomatic Mental Disorders:</u>

- F00- dementia in Alzheimer's disease
- F01- vascular dementia
- F04- organic amnesic syndrome, that wasn't caused by alcohol as well as other psychoactive drugs
- F06- other mental disorders due to brain damage and psychological disease.

Mental and Behavioural Disorders Due To Psychoactive Drugs Use The Codes F10-F19:

Basically, this is a range of mental conditions that are caused by the use of one or more psychoactive substances.

These drugs include:

- Alcohol
- Opioids
- Cocaine
- Sedatives or hypnotics
- And more…

Schizophrenia, schizotypal and delusional disorders: (F20-F29)

These codes can be broken down into:

F20- schizophrenia

F20.0- paranoid schizophrenia

F21- schizotypal disorders

Lastly, F30-F39 are mood disorders.

Finally, the USA and other countries use the Diagnostic and Statistical Manual (DSM-5) It's published by the American Psychological Association.

Biases in Diagnosis:

However, many biases affect diagnosis. For example:

- The sick role bias- when a doctor looks for something wrong with the patient because the patient came to them, so there must be something wrong.
- Confirmation bias- where doctors look for evidence to confirm their suspicions than evidence that doesn't.

And there is much, much more that can affect the reliability of diagnosis. But to drench your thirst for more here are two studies that show how unreliable diagnosis can be and a study showing the role of culture in diagnosis.

Rosenhan (1973):

8 mentally healthy people tried to get admission to a mental hospital.

In the interview, the patients said that they were hearing voices saying empty, hollow and thug. Apart from this, they told the truth about everything.

Upon admission, they acted normally and wanted to be discharged from the hospital.

They secretly took notes of their observations.

Results showed that seven of the 8 were admitted and were diagnosed with schizophrenia.

Took on average of 19 days for the patients to get out of the hospital via own means.

When discharged their schizophrenia was in remission.

None of the hospital staff thought they were healthy patients.

Normal behaviour was interpreted as symptoms of a disease.

In conclusion, psychiatrists lack the ability to tell the difference between a sane person and a disorder.

Critically Thinking:

A strength of the study is that the experiment was completed at a number of US hospitals so the results can be applied potentially to the whole country.

On the other hand, the study lacks temporal validity because the study was done back in the 1970s and since then our knowledge of disorders has improved, so the results probably wouldn't apply now.

Le-Repac (1980):

5 white and 4 Chinese American therapists were compared to see when shown a video of white and Chinese patients to see would their conclusions be the same.

They were tested on their definition of abnormality, empathetic ability and perception of the patient.

Results showed both cultures agreed on the concept of abnormality.

Americans were more accurate when predicting self-descriptive responses.

Americans thought Chinese patients were depressed and less socially poised.

Chinese thought Americans to be more disturbed.

Differences were down to therapists' own biases and world views.

Critically Thinking:

The study has strong internal validity; does the study measure what it intends to; because it shows that culture can affect a clinician's judgement.

However, the study doesn't use two distinctly

different cultures as both were American in whole or part. So, is it possible that the results would show a bigger or smaller gap of difference between other cultures?

PART TWO: DEPRESSION

CHAPTER 4: BIOLOGICAL EXPLANATION FOR DEPRESSION

Now, we're starting to get to what I call proper psychology and my favourite parts of psychology because to this and the next two chapters are some of the most interesting pieces of psychology.

As we start to explore the why and the reasons behind why Major Depressive Disorder develops.

Firstly, we are starting with a biological basis for MDD.

There are two theories for why MDD develops within the biological world. The first is called the serotonin hypothesis.

This theory states that MDD is caused by an imbalance of serotonin in the brain. Serotonin is a neurotransmitter associated with many functions in the body and it's sometimes referred to as the happiness chemical. As it's associated with happiness as well as well-being.[1]

There are two pieces of evidence supporting this hypothesis:

> • Supported by: certain drugs known to decrease serotonin are known to have depressive side effects.
> • Drugs that increase serotonin levels can relieve depression symptoms. Like: Selective Serotonin Reuptake Inhibitors (SSRIs)

However, a major criticism and a problem that I personally have with this theory is that once you take an SSRI the level of serotonin in your blood increases within an hour. However, depressive symptoms don't decrease until a month later.

Therefore, it begs the question: is it actually the increase in serotonin that cures your depression? Or does that increase start another bodily process and that process takes a month to finish and that process cures your depression?

I know that it sounds strange or not thought out but if the serotonin hypothesis is true, then surely your depression could be cured within an hour of you taking the SSRI as within that hour the serotonin

---

[1]

https://www.medicalnewstoday.com/kc/serotonin-facts-232248

imbalance is gone or reduced?

The Neurogenesis Hypothesis:

On the other hand, modern research has been focusing on the Neurogenesis theory of depression. The theory states that depression is the result of a lack of neuron birth in the hippocampus (this is the part of the brain responsible for emotion) and in other places in the brain that is related to serotonin, dopamine and norepinephrine.

In addition, cortisol appears to be the reason for this lack of neurogenesis. (the birth of neurons in the brain) Patients with MDD show a symptom called HPA-axis hyperactivity. This results in the over-secretion of cortisol. (too much cortisol is being released) This leads to reduced levels of serotonin as well as other neurotransmitters in the brain, including dopamine. This has been linked to depression. Demonstrating how complex the brain's chemistry is, and why the treatment for depression remains problematic. As we will explore later.

There are a few pieces of evidence that support this theory as well.

- Depressed people tend to have smaller hippocampi than the rest of the general population.
- Stress hormones are increased in MDD patients and this appears to stop neurogenesis

in the hippocampus, as shown in rodents and other primates.

- Finally, anti-depressants can increase neurogenesis in the hippocampus in rodents.[2]

Supporting Studies:

Caspi et al (2003):

The 5-HTT gene is responsible or the production of serotonin.

A longitudinal study of 1,037 children from New Zealand. Divided into three groups: people with two short alleles of the 5-HTT gene, one long and short alleles, two long alleles.

They were assessed from the age of 3 to 25.

A life history calendar was used to assess stressful life events.

Subjects were assessed for depression with an interview and information from someone who knew them well.

Results showed that there were no differences in the number of stressful life events.

People with two short alleles managed life events

---

[2]

https://www.thinkib.net/psychology/page/22460/biological-approach-to-depression

with more depressive symptoms.

Critically Thinking:

The study effective looks at the genetic argument for the serotonin hypothesis.

Nonetheless, this study does have ethical concerns. For example, the distress that knowing that you're genetically more likely to develop depression.

Therefore, the costs and benefits of research must always be calculated before the research is done.

Kendler et al (2006):

Over 42,000 twins were recruited for the study across a 60-year age span for the purpose of generational comparison.

They used a computer-assisted telephone interview that was conducted using DSM-4 criteria for MDD.

Informed consent was got before the interview. Trained interviewers were used with a lot of medical training to collect data.

The aim was to reach both pairs within a month.

Results showed prior studies got similar results. Heritability of depression is 38% on average.

Didn't differ very much across the generations.

No evidence was found that the shared environment was a factor in developing depression.

In conclusion, major depression is moderately inherited.

Critically Thinking:

The study is highly reliable as a number of studies have supported its findings that depression is about 37% inherited.

However, this study is open to population fallacy; were your sample does actually represent the general population; because most of the population aren't twins.

CHAPTER 5: COGNITIVE EXPLANATION FOR DEPRESSION

Moving to our next point of interest is how can our mental processes affect our chance of developing MDD.

Now the main theory of depression used for this type of explanation is: Beck (1967) and the theory states that cognition (mental processes) is the main reason behind depression and focuses on the impact that a change in automatic thoughts can have on behaviour. The theory focuses on:

- The cognitive triad- negative beliefs about the self, the world and the future. These influence the automatic thoughts to be pessimistic.
- Negative schema- the negative beliefs about themselves become generalize and people start to think negatively about everything that happens to them.

- Faulty thinking patterns- people think and make illogical conclusions because of how they process information is biased.

Personally, I do quite like the theory because if you know someone with depression as I did then you can see some of this theory in real life.

In addition, I think that it's a reasonably easy theory to follow.

But let's put this theory into context, according to this theory a depression is caused by:

(I know some the examples are poor)

- The cognitive triad- this can be demonstrated when a depressed person says things. Like: "I'm useless," or "Oh the world is falling apart so what's the point of living?"
- Negative schemas- as demonstrated by this: "Oh I failed in art so I'm never going to pass any subjects, go to university and I'm just going to be a failure in life,"
- Faulty thinking patterns- this could be shown in a setting when researching a holiday to the most beautiful place ever and there was a 0.5% chance of a terror attack. "Oh no, I can't go there I'm going to die,"

While that last example wasn't the best. It shows how illogical conclusions can be made because of a bias towards the negative.

Supporting studies:

This first study shows how having a negative thinking style can affect depression.

Alloy, Abramson and Francis (1999):

Quasi-experiment and longitudinal study for 5.5 years with a questionnaire and structured interviews.

Freshmen were given a questionnaire to determine their cognitive style and they were split into two groups based on the results.

High risk; the negative cognitive style; believed that negative life events were cataphoric and the results meant that they were flawed and worthless.

During the first 2.5 years, high-risk people were more likely to develop symptoms of major depression. (17% versus 1%)

High-risk people were more likely to have suicidal thoughts and behaviour (28% versus 13%)

In conclusion, negative cognitive style can lead to the development of major depression.

Critically thinking:

This study was a longitudinal study, so this allowed the researchers to show the effects of a negative thinking style over time.

Yet it was a quasi-experiment without a clear independent variable and the dependent variable, so it can't be said if the study has strong internal validity; does the study measure what it intended to; as it wasn't clear what the study was measuring.

Caseras et al (2007):

Quasi-experiment with eye-tracking technology

Using the Beck Depression Inventory, the subjects were assessed for depressive symptoms and then split into two groups. Depressed and non-depressed.

Then the subjects were shown 32 pictures paired with a positive, neutral and negative stimuli and each picture was shown for 3 seconds.

Using eye-tracking technology, the researchers measured what stimuli the subject first focused on and how long they focused on it before they switched to another stimulus.

Results showed that depressed people have an attention bias for the negative stimuli because once they looked at the negative stimuli, they found it hard to move onto another stimulus.

Critically Thinking:

The study used a large sample bias so the findings can be applied to large groups of people as we know that this trend of behaviour is shown by several people.

However, this is a reductionist way of thinking. A way of thinking that tries to find a single cause for depression without thinking of other factors and more holistic research that considers biological, cognitive and social factors of depression needs to be done.

Summary:

Beck (1967) theory focuses on the cognitive triad, negative schemas and faulty thinking processes.

Alloy, Abramson and Francis (1999) shows how a negative thinking style can lead to depression.

Caseras et al (2007) found that depressed people have an attention bias to negative stimuli.

CHAPTER 6: SOCIAL EXPLANATION FOR DEPRESSION

Personally, this section is the least interesting for me because while I fully know that social factors DO play a role in depression and believe me I know.

I think that this section is really common sense about what social factors can cause depression and I prefer to learn and know the more theoretical content of psychology.

So as there's no theory to talk about. Let's quickly run through some factors that could cause depression.

These are the factors that Brown and Harris (1978) found that could increase the development of depression.

- Having 3 or more children
- Lack of intimate relationships
- Lack of employment
- Loss of mother

Supporting studies:

Kivela et al (1996):

Quasi-experimental, longitudinal study

A study was completed in 1984-85 on depression of over 1,500 elderly Finnish people.

Those that were not depressed were interviewed and reassessed in a follow-up study in 1989-1990.

Through questionnaires, certain life events and social variables that occurred during 1984-1989 were assessed.

Depressed and non-depressed people were compared.

Results showed that in 1989-90 8.2% of men were depressed and 9.3% of women were depressed.

Powerful predictors for men were: poor relationship and negative change with Spouse, moving into intuitional care and loss of mother under twenty.

Powerful predictors for women were: loss of father under 20, low religious activity and worsening relationship with neighbours.

In conclusion, social factors and changes in social ties can be predictors in developing depression at old age.

Critically Thinking:

While the study effectively shows how elderly people can get depressed because of social factors. There is probably a lack of temporal validity; how valid the results are because of time; because Finland like the rest of the world has gone through the cultural and social change since this experiment was done. Therefore, can the results still be valid considering this social change over time?

Unless the experiment is redone, we will not know.

Rosenquist, Fowler and Christakis (2011):

You will find this study interesting!

Statical analysis of social networks and longitudinal study.

Participants were taken from an earlier study in 1948 in Framingham and the researchers took the information in order to keep track of these people in case they were needed again.

A questionnaire for depression was done three times between 1981-2001.

Rosenquist, Fowler and Christakis computerized and analysed the data in 2011.

Results showed that people up to 3 degrees of

separation could be affected because:

Subjects were 93% more likely to get depressive symptoms if they were in direct contact with a depressed person.

43% for two degrees

37% for three degrees

Critically Thinking:

The study is numbers based so the results have a good scientific basis to support.

But the data of this study is fairly old and because we live in an ever-changing and developing world. How do we know if the results are still valid?

Is it possible the results are higher or lower in today's society with the increased use of social media and other factors?

The problem with social research is that it needs to be redone about every ten years because of the fact that we live in a changing world.

Summary:

Kivela et al (1996) shows that there are a number of factors involved in depression in elderly people.

Rosenquist, Fowler and Christakis (2011) shows how depression can spread through a social network.

PART THREE: ANXIETY, OBSESSIVE COMPULSIVE DISORDERS & SCHIZOPHRENIA

CHAPTER 7: ANXIETY DISORDERS

After looking at depression, I thought that it would be good to look at some other psychological conditions that people can develop.

Personally, I loved this lecture at university because I love learning but it gave me the chance to learn about other types of mental conditions as well.

What are Anxiety Disorders?

This is a group of disorders that are distinguished by feelings of wrong and intense stress as well as when the sufferer makes attempts to deal with these feelings. Their methods are disruptive and largely unsuccessful.

Unfortunately, anxiety disorders are moderately common as the lifetime prevalence; how common the condition is in a population; of this condition is 29% (Kessler et al, 2005) and it's more common in women than men. (Bresula, Chilcoal, Kessler and Davis,

1999)

In addition, the term anxiety disorders can be broken down into a lot of different sub-categories.

Phobias:

Phobias are a great subcategory to start off with as they're well-known and television programmes love to use them.

But what actually are phobias?

A phobia is a very intense and irrational fear that is usually paired with great determination as well as an effort to avoid the object.

Such as: if you have a phobia of spiders then you would not only have an intense fear of spiders, but you would do everything in your power to avoid them as well.

Additionally, specific phobias are any disorder that is characterised by an extreme as well as an irrational fear of a certain object or situation. Like: flying, spiders or snakes.

Overall, the prevalence of any specific phobia is 13% (Kessler et al, 2005) and women are twice as likely to have a specific phobia than men. (Bourdon et al, 1988)

Social Phobia/ Social Anxiety Disorder:

I once knew a girl who suffered from Social Anxiety Disorder and it was interesting from a psychological perspective; at least; to talk to her about social situations because she hated them. She hated being watched, judged and anything to do with being social.

Yet she was very social with certain people who she knew wouldn't judge her.

Moving onto the content, people with social phobias are very fearful about being watched or judged by others.

Interestingly, it is not only negative perception or evaluation that is fearful but positive evaluation as well. (Weeks, Heinberg, Rodebaugh and Norton, 2008)

That fact makes this disorder very interesting because it's natural to assume that the person would be concerned about negative evaluations. Like:

"She looks awful,"

"What is he doing? What an idiot?"

"The gym obviously isn't working for them!"

Yet it makes almost no sense for them to be concerned about positive evaluations. Such as:

"He's great to talk to,"

"That's an amazing piece of work!"

"I love your cake, Sarah!"

Nonetheless, one of the possible reasons for why sufferers of this condition might hate positive evaluations is because it sets a standard and then they become fearful of them missing the standard in the future. Leading to people judging them because they failed this time.

Putting that into practice using the cake example, Sarah could make a great cake this time but as her friends think she's an amazing cook now. She could become anxious over the thought of failing to bake another amazing cake, and her friends judging her for her failure.

Furthermore, men and women are affected equally by this disorder as well as it typically manifests itself in childhood or adolescence. (Robins and Regier, 1991)

This is a very interesting fact and it probably explains the behaviour of the girl that I knew.

Interestingly, sometimes a social phobia is limited to only one situation; like speaking in groups; whilst in other cases, social phobias are widespread or generalised to many or all social situations.

Going back to the girl I knew, she hated meeting strangers and talking to them, but she was fine being the centre of attention for people that she knew.

Another downside of Social Anxiety Disorder:

In addition, to the suffering, the panic and the awful feelings associated with this condition.

When forced into situations, people that suffer from social phobia may use drugs or alcohol to 'fortify' themselves. This increases the risk of alcohol and substance abuse or dependency. (Pollack, 2001)

Which leads to many more problems for the individual.

Panic Disorders:

This is another type of disorder that I've accounted in my life as I've had one or two friends that suffer from panic attacks as well as panic disorders. Especially, in social situations.

What are Panic Disorders?

This is a type of anxiety disorder that can be characterised by repeated or debilitating panic attacks.

Panic attacks are a sudden episode of horrific bodily symptoms. Like: choking, chest pains and distress.

All anxiety disorders involve panic attacks, yet a panic disorder involves panic attacks that come out the blue.

For example, the girl I knew that suffered from Social Anxiety Disorder had panic attacks in social situations and only those situations.

Nevertheless, a sufferer of a panic disorder would suffer from a panic attack in any situation.

Finally, panic disorders are found in 5% women and 2% men. (Barlow, 2002)

Generalised Anxiety Disorder:

Whilst, people with phobias and panic attacks suffer massively and their lives can be very disturbed. Both of these conditions are limited as without the stimulus or trigger these people can function almost 'normally'

This doesn't apply to people with Generalised Anxiety Disorder because these people aren't anxious about a particular thing. Instead, their anxiety is continuous and severe.

This disorder is relatively common as it has a prevalence of 6% (Kessler et al 2005) as well as it's twice as likely to be found in women than men.

An example of Generalised Anxiety Disorder is: "I'm so nervous about making a mistake at work I take all my reports home to rewrite them the night before I'm suppose to hand them in" (White, 1999, p.72)

People with generalised anxiety disorder worry about everything and anything, as well as these people, feel inadequate, can't concentrate, are oversensitive and may sometimes suffer from insomnia.

According to Rickels and Ryan (2001), these behaviours can be accompanied by irregular breathing, chronic diaherria, rapid heart rate and excessive sweating.

Personally, I feel so sorry for these people as Generalized Anxiety Disorder can be very debilitating and stop you from enjoying life.

CHAPTER 8: OBSESSIVE COMPULSION DISORDER AND WHAT CAUSES ANXIETY DISORDERS?

Another interesting anxiety disorder that has been popularised by the media is the mental condition Obsessive Compulsive Disorder, also known as OCD, and I write this during the COVID-19 pandemic and a minor of the public believe that COVID-19 will cause them to develop OCD. As they will become obsessed with washing their hands.

Now, this is unlikely to happen because OCD isn't caused by obsessively doing an action as that's a symptom of the condition as well as there are other factors involved in the development of OCD.

What is Obsessive-Compulsive Disorder?

This disorder involves a person having an obsession. These are recurring thoughts and ritualistic behaviours that can potentially be used to deal with an obsession.

For example, if your obsession is to be clean then the behaviour could be to wash your hands constantly.

Obsession compulsive disorder affects approximately 2% of the population at some point in their lives. (Kessler et al,2005) as well as it affects both sexes equally and it's very serious.

As a result, if it is left untreated then it tends to get worse over time as well as it can be accompanied by depressive episodes. (Barlow, 1988)

What Causes Obsessive Compulsive Disorder and other Anxiety Disorders?

Genetic risk factors:

Always biological factors are involved in the development of anxiety disorders and twin studies show a clear inheritability for anxiety disorders, and pairs of identical twins are much more likely to get an anxiety disorder. If one of them has it compared to non-identical or normal siblings. (Hettema, Neale and Kendler, 2001)

Although, as there are a lot of different genes that are thought to be involved in anxiety disorders. It's hard to narrow down which gene causes these types of disorders.

In addition, there's even some evidence suggesting that there are different inheritable pathways for different aspects of OCD. (Leckman, Zhang, Alsobroo and Pauls, 2001) for example, hoarding or washing hands.

Nonetheless, it must be remembered that genetics factors alone don't cause a disorder. As a result, it is the genetic vulnerability that is exposed to a type of trigger or stressor that causes the disorder. (Binder et al, 2008)

Brain Bases:

Recently, a number of functional imaging studies have found some interesting results.

For example, the brain regions that are responsible for fear learning are highly active in people with phobias. (Etkin and Wager, 2007; Goldin et al, 2009)

These findings suggest that people with anxiety disorders learn fears easier than other people. Possibly explaining why they are anxious or fearful of certain things but other people are not.

Psychological Factors:

Finally, there are always psychological reasons for why a condition develops. Including:

- Experiences- these negative experiences can make a person fearful of a similar situation in case the experience happens again.

For example, if someone experiences embarrassment or bullying after talking in a group. Then they can become fearful of talking in groups in case they experience the bullying or embarrassment again.

- Trauma- very similar to the reason above but to a more extreme degree.

Hopefully, after this short section, you can start to appreciate the complexity and severity of anxiety disorders and how impactful they can be on someone's life.

But how are they treated?

How is depression treated?

After looking at Schizophrenia that will be the question we investigate.

CHAPTER 9: SCHIZOPHRENIA

Whenever a person thinks of a mental condition or the mentally ill; I hate that term; they are bound to think of Schizophrenia. As it's constantly used in the media, TV and other ways that have captured the public's imagination and interest in this unfortunate condition.

Truth be told, I'm quite interested in this condition as I find the idea of hearing voices, the theories behind the causes of Schizophrenia and more to be extremely interesting.

However, as this book is mainly focused on depression, I'm only going to be quickly talking about the interesting condition known as Schizophrenia.

<u>What is Schizophrenia?</u>

To put it bluntly, Schizophrenia is a group of mental disorders that are characterised by being withdrawn, delusions, hallucinations and disturbances of thought.

I should note here that the hallucinations that Schizophrenics suffer from can be both auditory; so they hear things; and visual. Meaning that they see things.

How Common is Schizophrenia?

As I spoke about in my Forensic Psychology book, the media has a tendency to make people think that crimes and mental conditions are a lot more common than they are in reality.

However, the prevalence rate; how common a condition is; for Schizophrenia is very interesting because whilst the prevalence of schizophrenia is about 1%. There are a lot of geographical variations that aren't well understood.

For example, the rates of Schizophrenia are higher in Croatia and the western half of Ireland compared to the quite low rate found in Papua New Guinea.

That fact, I find very interesting because it poses so many great questions for research. For example:

- Why do the differences exist?
- Is there something about the Papua New Guinea culture that makes Schizophrenia less likely?

- What is it about Western Ireland that increases the chance of getting Schizophrenia? Age? Diet?

Typically, schizophrenia is diagnosed in early adulthood or late adolescence, this tends to be earlier for males than females. (Jabensky and Cole, 1997) also, men tend to develop worse forms of the condition compared to women.

Can You Recover from Schizophrenia?

As of yet, there is, unfortunately, no cure for Schizophrenia and the news gets worse.

Sadly, the chance of people recovering from schizophrenia isn't encouraging.

As a result, Andreasen and Black (1996) and Cutting (1986) tracked 200 people in the United States with schizophrenia and they showed over 30 years:

- 20% of them were doing well.
- 45% were incapacitated.
- 66% never married.
- 58% had never worked.

Unfortunately, these studies merely highlight how awful Schizophrenia can be to people as it can severely impact your life.

Despite the rather grim recovery chances, I just

explained. There are a few treatment options for schizophrenia but I must stress there is no cure so all these treatment options do is lessen the symptoms of the condition.

One treatment option for schizophrenia is to prescribe antipsychotic or neuroleptic drugs. These drugs block dopamine synapses and prevent them from releasing excess dopamine. I'll explain why this is important in a moment.

Nonetheless, prolonged use of anti-psychotic drugs could lead to the client developing a type of movement disorder called tardive Dyskinesia. This is presumably where the horrid term "retard" comes from. No one should ever be called that.

Although, second-generation drugs relieve the symptoms without producing the tardive Dyskinesia. Yet these drugs don't improve the client's overall quality of life any better than the original drugs.

Again, sadly the prospects of recovery from schizophrenia is a depressing read.

Additional Statistics:

According to Saha et al (2005), there is a 7:5 male to female ratio for schizophrenia. Making it more common in males than females and it tends to be more severe and has an earlier onset for males.

With the average onset of schizophrenia being 18 in men and 25 in women.

Nonetheless, after a heavy section, I want to mention a quick funny story because back when I was doing psychology in 6th Form (High school for the rest of the world) I had a psychology teacher who told us she was relieved when she turned 21 (she was told that was onset age) and she did not have schizophrenia.

She described it to us as she was delighted and overwhelmed with joy.

What are the Symptoms of Schizophrenia?

Before I dive into the symptoms, I want to highlight like most mental health conditions, the symptoms can vary dramatically from person to person.

Also, schizophrenia can be acute with a sudden onset and good prospects of recovery, or chronic with a gradual onset and extremely poor prospects of recovery.

In short, the symptoms of Schizophrenia can be described as a deteriorating ability to function in everyday life plus two or more of the following:

- Hallucinations
- Delusion

- Movement disorder
- Inappropriate emotional expressions
- Thought disorder

Positive Symptoms:

These are symptoms that are not evident in healthy people.

For example, delusions; these are incorrect beliefs that are strongly maintained despite strong evidence to the contrary.

According to Cutting (1995), 90% of people with schizophrenia suffer from delusions.

Hallucinations are another positive symptom and according to functional brain imaging, research has shown increased activation in primary auditory regions in the temporal lobe. (Lennox, Park, Medley, Morris and Jones, 2000)

This finding suggests that schizophrenic people have auditory hallucinations; hear voices; that are as vivid and real to them as real human voices.

Personally, I find that this is another extremely interesting fact because I believe that it's amazing to know that the brain honestly believes that it's hearing real voices.

However, it isn't.

So, I'm very interested to know why.

Negative Symptoms:

These symptoms are a group of symptoms that take away from the patient's state of well-being.

For example, some negative symptoms that Schizophrenics suffer from include:

- Flattening- staring into space and little emotional expression.
- Catatonic
- People with schizophrenia suffer from anhedonia. This is where they don't find pleasure in activities that healthy people do.

Furthermore, Gard et al (2007) found that anhedonia corresponded with lower levels of goal-oriented behaviour.

- Withdrawal from others is another major symptom of Schizophrenia. (Tarbox, and Pogue-Geile, 2008)

CHAPTER 10: WHAT CAUSES SCHIZOPHRENIA?

There are a lot of different causes of Schizophrenia and there is no one cause so everything below; for lack of a better term; interacts together to cause the condition.

The Dopamine Hypothesis:

This hypothesis was proposed by Meltzer & Stahl (1976) and they thought schizophrenia was caused by excess activity of dopamine synapses in certain areas of the brain.

This I think is interesting since we tend to associate dopamine with positive behaviours so the thought that dopamine can do us harm is weird at first. Yet in Biological Psychology I discuss how much damage various neurotransmitters can do to us.

So, this hypothesis is interesting, to say the least.

Furthermore, this hypothesis is supported by several key pieces of evidence. For example, drugs that provoke a similar state to schizophrenia (like amphetamines) increase stimulation of dopamine synapses. (Martinez et al, 2007) Meaning there's a link between stimulation of the synapses and schizophrenia.

Additionally, drugs that alleviate schizophrenia block postsynaptic dopamine receptors. (Dimitilis & Shanker, 2016) and drugs that are the most effective at blocking dopamine receptors also are the most effective against schizophrenia.

Overall, this evidence provides good evidence for this theory and I quite like the hypothesis since it's logical and it makes sense.

However, there is evidence against this hypothesis. Such as: drugs that block postsynaptic dopamine receptors don't always alleviate schizophrenia for all patients, and there are inconsistent results about the measurements of dopamine or its metabolites.

On the whole, I want to add that this hypothesis is quite good but it's similar to the serotonin hypothesis in depression. Because it's just a biological factor and it doesn't take the cognitive or social factors into account.

The Glutamate hypothesis:

Another biological hypothesis for the cause of schizophrenia is the Glutamate hypothesis proposed by Moghaddam & Javitt (2012). This propose schizophrenia is partially caused by a lack of Glutamate activity.

This is a problem because Glutamate inhibits dopamine release so this hypothesis builds upon the dopamine hypothesis and explains why the excess dopamine levels occur.

Saying that the lack of Glutamate activity occurs because Phencyclidine blocks the glutamate synapses. Preventing it from being released into the synaptic gap. (Murray, 2002) as well as Schizophrenia is associated with lower than normal release of glutamate and fewer receptors in the prefrontal cortex and hippocampus (Harrison et al., 2003)

Leading to this interaction of both positive and negative symptoms of schizophrenia. Especially, in people already predisposed to the condition.

Overall, I believe these two hypotheses largely build upon one another and these are good explanations for the biological explanation of schizophrenia.

Genetic and Prenatal Factors:

For a long time, schizophrenia has been known to run in families. As supported by Andreasen and Black (1996) as it found that a sibling of a person with schizophrenia is four times more likely to develop schizophrenia than the general population.

Nevertheless, there are always problems with the research.

However, whilst the evidence above could be perceived to be down to environmental factors. The results from twin studies show that the likelihood of identical twins developing schizophrenia if the other twin has it is between 41%- 65% and 6%-28% for non-identical twins. (Cardno and Gottesman, 2000)

In addition, genetics aren't the only possible cause of schizophrenia as prenatal influences; influences during pregnancy; can cause schizophrenia as well.

Such as prenatal influences include a diminished supply of oxygen to the brain as well as a number of prenatal infections can contribute to schizophrenia.

Furthermore, the evidence suggests that schizophrenia is a neurodevelopmental disorder. Meaning that from a young age the brain doesn't develop as it's meant to; also this means that schizophrenia could be detected in early adulthood.

Finally, stress is another contributing factor to the development of schizophrenia as explained in the introduction. Stress can trigger a genetic disposition to cause a condition.

This explains the higher prevalence of schizophrenia in people with a lower socioeconomic status.

Other biological causes of schizophrenia include:

- Poor nutrition for mother
- Extreme maternal stress during pregnancy
- Season of birth effect
- Viral infections and influenzas.
- Premature birth, low birth weight and complications in delivery.

Neurodevelopmental Hypothesis:

In addition, to the biological causes of this condition, a new line of thinking is starting to develop to consider there might be a neurodevelopmental cause of schizophrenia. Yet it isn't firmly established currently.

For instance, some psychologists believe damage to an infant's dorsolateral prefrontal cortex could be a factor. Since at one year old there is little effect of the brain lesion, as well as infants perform as well as undamaged monkeys when performing tasks.

However, at 2 years old, the effects of the lesion are clear and the 2-year-old infant performs a lot worse than undamaged monkeys.

PART FOUR: TREATMENT

CHAPTER 11: INTRODUCTION TO TREATMENT

After looking at various mental health conditions and their causes, we're now going to be looking at the very important topic of treatment.

As a subject, I truly love treatment because as a species we have come such a long way; as outlined in the introduction; in terms of our understanding of mental conditions. That thankfully we can now treat people with varying success.

Of course, I know that we still have a long way to go in terms of treating a lot of conditions but at least we can help a lot of people suffering from a range of conditions.

But first of all, why is treatment important?

Why bother treating people?

What does treatment provide people with?

In short, treatment for mental conditions offers people the chance to live a 'normal' life and enjoy life to the extent that a clinically normal person can.

For more information on the importance of treatment, please check out: www.connorwhiteley.net/clinicalpsychology

Who provides this Treatment?

This isn't a straight forward answer as a wide range of professionals can deliver treatment for people but in this introduction, we'll be focusing on Clinical Psychologists.

These are psychologists that are specially trained in treating, assessing and helping people with mental conditions. That's the short answer.

As previously mentioned, Clinical psychologists assess people for mental disorders and they can deliver psychological treatment, and they work in a range of settings. Such as schools, clinics and private practices.

Other professions that can deliver treatment for mental conditions with a simple explanation includes:

- Psychiatrists- in essence, a psychologist that can prescribe drugs.

- Neurologist- a profession that has great knowledge of the brain's functionality and how it impacts our behaviour and functions.
- Mental health counsellors- someone who you can talk to. To help you with your difficulties.

Interestingly when it comes to the professionals delivering the treatment, the more experienced professionals aren't always more effective than less experienced professionals. (McFall, 2006) and credentials doesn't guarantee therapeutic success either. (Blatt, Sanislow, Zuroff and Pilkonis, 1996)

Suggesting that who the therapist is and how they match the patient's needs is more important than experience and degrees.

Note: of course, the professional still needs to have qualifications and experience to be effective but themselves as a person and what they are like with their clients is also very important.

For example, 'clicking' with your therapist or client is very important to the therapy's success.

Another interesting fact about patients and treatment is that sometimes people seek treatment not only to relieve them of the pain of diagnosable conditions; like depression; but subsyndromal conditions as well.

These subsyndromal conditions are an instance

where a person has a mental condition but not to the intensity, frequency or other criteria for it to be diagnosed. (Ratey and Johnstone, 1997)

For instance, they may suffer from Major Depression but not enough to be officially diagnosed.

Therefore, they are still suffering from the condition, so they need the treatment as well as help.

Hence, why they go to therapy still despite not having an 'official' mental condition.

CHAPTER 12: APPROACHES TO PSYCHOLOGICAL TREATMENT

Before, we dive into the ways how psychological treatments can be used to treat depression. I think that it's vital that we learn the different types and approaches that can be used in psychological treatment as psychotherapy comes in the form of over 500 types (Eisner, 2000)

That's a lot!

So, let us begin…

Psychodynamic Approach:

I think that it's fair to say that these types of treatment are the best well-known as these types of therapy are popular on television.

But what actually is the psychodynamic approach to treatment?

These treatment types are based on the beliefs of Freud who believed that a patient's illness was caused by an internal conflict that developed in their childhood.

Subsequently, by adulthood, the patient would build a range of defences to deal with this conflict. Yet these defences would prevent them from seeing the world clearly, causing a range of problems that showed themselves as psychological symptoms.

In order to treat this person, Freud believed that the patient needed to work through their problem. Allowing them to integrate their thought as well as feelings into a cohesive order. This would allow them to overcome these maladaptive behaviours that don't let them see the world clearly.

It's an interesting idea and as I talk about in my Cognitive Psychology book it isn't how the unconscious works but it's a great idea.

Modern versions of this approach include interpersonal therapy.

This is a form of therapy that focuses on helping the patient to understand how they interact with others so they can learn better ways to interact as well as communicate.

Humanistic Approach:

However, psychologists that take the humanistic approach criticize the psychodynamic approach as they believe that the psychodynamic approach focuses on basic urges too much, instead of meaning.

This has led to them proposing several types of their own therapies that make the client take responsibility for their actions and life. In order to live life to its fullest.

For example, Roger's (a very important figure in clinical psychology) client rental therapy is where the therapist doesn't question or direct the patient instead they listen intensively. To create a positive atmosphere where the client can learn to accept themselves for who they are.

According to Rogers (1980), unconditional positive regard and empathic understanding are all very important in therapy.

Personally, I'm very interested in this model or type of therapy because I love the idea of helping people to accept themselves. Instead of telling them that something is wrong with them and making them change themselves.

Of course, this wouldn't work for all mental conditions but for some conditions, this type of therapy could be great.

Other types of Humanistic Therapy Include:

- Motivational- enhancement therapy (Miller and Rollnicj, 2002)

This therapy is a brief, non-confrontational client centred therapy that is designed to challenge specific problematic behaviours.

- Gestalt therapy- associated with Fitz Perls.

This therapy aims to increase self-awareness as well as self-acceptance to help the patient or client fit their inconsistent selves into one cohesive self.

In other words, this Gestalt therapy helps a person to accept themselves and gain awareness of the different aspects of the Self. Leading to acceptance of all of these different aspects.

Behaviourist Approach:

This approach to treatment focuses on conditioning as the cause of mental disorders as well as you need to break the associations between the stimuli and the fear as seen in phobias.

For example, exposure therapy is an example of this approach as exposure therapy aims to create a new connection. This is where the stimulus creates a response that displaces the fear due to its incompatibility.

In simple terms, the new connection replaces the fear that the person has as this new connection doesn't elicit a fear response. Like the old connection does.

In order to start the therapy, the patient must create an anxiety hierarchy. Meaning that they create a sequence of events from least to most fear-provoking.

For instances, the patient is first conditioned against the least fear provoking before becoming counter conditioned against the more fear-provoking situation.

Note: this is all imagined.

A practical example of this could be that a person is fearful of spiders could imagine that a spider is in the room.

This would be the least fear-provoking.

Before imagining that the spider is going down their arm away from them and so on.

However, sometimes this counter-conditioning must be applied in the real world. Such as: visiting a tall building or touching spiders.

This is called: In Vivo Desensitization.

Operant Conditioning Techniques:

This treatment involves the idea of reinforcement were the patients are rewarded for desirable behaviours and punished for undesirable behaviour.

One example of this treatment is a token economy. Where the patient gets rewarded with tokens and these tokens can be adjusted over time to shape the behaviour of the patient. Then the patient can exchange these tokens for tangible rewards. Like: snacks, watching TV or books.

For example, the patient could get a token for getting out of bed in the morning but after a week it could change. Making the patient have to get up and get dressed before they receive the token.

This idea of the token economy, I quite like because if you suffer from depression then even the thought of getting out of bed is difficult. Therefore, having a reward can be helpful in performing this seemingly impossible task.

Modelling:

Another powerful therapy is modelling where the patient watches the therapist's or another person's behaviour to learn new skills.

In addition, this modelling isn't limited to

physical actions as it can be applied to thought processes as well.

For example, the therapist thinks aloud to solve a common problem, so the patient a new skill for a similar situation. (Kendall, 1990)

Integrated Therapies:

Eclecticism is an approach to treatment that pulls together and weaves multiple types as well as forms of therapy together. (Beitman, Goldfriend and Norrcross, 1989)

An example of this eclecticism is Linehan's Dialectical Behaviour Therapy (DBT) for borderline personality disorder because this therapy weaves the cognitive, behavioural and humanistic as well as psychodynamic approaches together.

This approach to therapy is great because it offers the therapist flexibility to propose and follow enquires and back away from ineffective approaches and this allows the therapist to find the different causes of the disorder. As different approaches target different causes.

In my opinion, this is a great idea for therapists because I was talking to my Lecturer at University about this and she completely agreed with me when I said that this is a great idea. As surely if a therapist only uses one type of therapy or approach to treatment then this can harm the effectiveness of the treatment.

In addition, she added as well that in the United Kingdom at least when you're doing your clinical placement also known as your doctoral training. You train in three different models or types of therapy.

For example, I think that my lecturer trained in Cognitive Behavioural Therapy, Psychodynamic Therapy and Systemic Therapy.

For more information on these types of therapies, please check out my Clinical Psychology book.

Shared Problem Groups:

This approach to therapy looks at bringing people together who have the same problem allowing them to offer advice and learn that they aren't alone.

For example, Alcohol Anonymous, Gambling Anonymous and Narcotics Anonymous.

Therapy Groups:

In groups, trained therapists can use a wide range of techniques to treat the group. Such as: behavioural or psychodynamic.

Nonetheless, the treatment truly begins when the patient learns that they aren't any different from others facing the same problem.

The additional benefits of the group are belongingness, encouragement as well as support.

All these benefits are important to the overall success of the treatment.

Finally, these group treatments can be seen to great effect in a variety of situations. For example, drugs and as explored in my Forensic Psychology book sex offenders.

Couple and Family Therapy:

Sadly, some couples and families need therapy because of various factors. Leading them to try and hopefully recover in therapy.

However, couple as well as family therapy is unique as these therapists view the family as a system of emotions with the feeling and thoughts all the people in the system influencing it heavily.

Meaning that if one person has a problem in the family or couple then this problem creates a ricochet effect throughout the entire system.

Another term for this 'systems' idea is systemic therapy.

Interestingly, according to Miklovitz (2007), a family-level intervention can decrease the relapse rate of people suffering from bipolar disorder.

In other words, if you address the family issues that could be causing or maintaining bipolar disorder then you can greatly help the sufferer of bipolar.

<u>Departing Note:</u>

I hope that you've found this slightly longer than usual chapter interesting and it's opened your mind to the many interesting types of psychotherapy and approaches that therapists can take to treat mental conditions.

Hopefully, in the future, I will dedicate a book to each of these approaches or types of therapy.

CHAPTER 13: BIOLOGICAL TREATMENT

So now that we understand how MDD is caused, we can start the last leg of our journey and start to understand how mental conditions are treated. Starting with depression.

Therefore, we already know biology can be used to treat depression because of anti-depressants. These are drugs that tend to increase serotonin levels in the body and then a month later your symptoms start to go.

(Remember Selective Serotonin Reuptake Inhibitors from earlier?)

Although there is another kind of anti-depressant, I want to mention in the book. This is called: Tricyclics. Two examples of these drugs are Impramine and Tofranil.

Tricyclics work just like SSRIs in terms of

preventing the reuptake of neurotransmitters to boost their concentration in the synaptic gap and restore the chemical imbalance.

Although, the unique feature of Tricyclics is this type of anti-depressant is these drugs work on dopamine and norepinephrine as well as serotonin.

This is done by the anti-depressant blocking histamine and acetylcholine receptors and some sodium channels.

Predictable Side Effects:

As always, I like to add in my opinion and I wouldn't like to have tricyclics if I ever got depression. The reason simply being tricyclics have the questionable side effects of heart problems and dry mouth.

Personally, I do not want to have heart problems so I would hope to avoid tricyclics if I got depression.

Monoamine Oxidase Inhibitors:

Moving onto another type of biological treatment for depression, I'm going to talk about Monoamine Oxidase Inhibitors (MOI). Since these are a bit different.

MOI is an enzyme that metabolises catecholamines (various class of neurochemicals including stress neurochemicals) and serotonin and this inhibits the concentrations of the catecholamines. This restores the chemical imbalance.

Finally, MOIs are only prescribed if SSRIs and tricyclics prove to be ineffective in treating the client's depression.

That's basically all you need to know about the biological treatment, as well as drugs focus on restoring the chemical imbalance in the body.

Elkin et al (1989):

250 patients were assigned into a placebo, medication, CBT or interpersonal psychotherapy group.

Treatment in groups went for 16 weeks.

Results showed that all 3 active groups outperformed the placebo group.

For mild and moderate depression there was no significant difference in the results for the three groups.

However, there was a clear advantage for medication over psychotherapy for serve depression.

In conclusion, drugs are more effective than psychological treatment for severe depression

Critically Thinking:

While the study was well controlled as other groups were used to compare the performances of drugs.

The study could lack temporal validity because since 1989 drugs have come a long way and have improved. Thus, it is possible that the results could be different now because of the advances in medical drugs?

Kirsch et al (2002):

A meta-analysis of published and unpublished data from clinical trials on antidepressants.

Results show that 82% of the effects of antidepressants are the same as the placebo.

In conclusion, when published and unpublished data are combined, they fail to show the effectiveness of antidepressants.

Critically Thinking:

This study manages to get around publication bias; were only positive studies tend to get published; as they used both published and unpublished data, so the results are a fair and balanced look at the antidepressants' effectiveness.

However, a meta-analysis can be flawed if there

are studies used with the analysis that is an outlier compared to the other studies used. In other words, the study doesn't include, or the results are very different from the other studies included. This can end up skewing the results of the analysis and causing the wrong conclusion to be drawn.

Therefore, it's important that only studies that are related and suitable are used in the analysis.

Summary:

Elkin et al (1989) shows medication is best for treating serve depression.

Kirsch et al (2012) shows that the overall effectiveness of antidepressants is there they aren't effective.

CHAPTER 14: OTHER BIOLOGICAL TREATMENT

Before we dive into another interesting area of psychological treatment to treat depression and other mental conditions, I wanted to quickly talk about some other ways that biology can be used to treat people.

As some of the methods are logical and common whereas others are... unusual and controversial.

Pharmacological or Drug Treatment:

This is definitely one of the common ways of treating depression and this is why I have a problem with psychiatry over psychology as in my experience they prefer to solve a problem with drugs. Instead of trying to find the psychological or social reasons for depression or another condition.

For example, if a person is suffering from depression and their main cause of stress is a bad home life and the sufferer may not even realise this is the main cause of the condition for them.

How will giving them anti-depressants fix this main cause?

Whereas in certain forms of psychotherapy, a psychologist would want to find out about the home life and other factors that can cause their depression. In an effort to treat the depression holistically.

Even if my interpretation of psychiatry is slightly bias, I hope that that story has got you thinking about the fact that not all psychological conditions can be solved using drugs.

Anyway, over the years as our understanding of mental conditions have increased, our ability to produce drug treatments for mental conditions has increased as well.

Additionally, drugs treatments have had an impact on mental health care as they allow people to be treated for illnesses without being hospitalised.

These treatments involve psychotropic drugs that control or moderate the symptoms of some mental disorders.

This feature of drug treatment has the great benefit of freeing up hospital beds, resources as well as staff to treat other people. In turn, decreasing the strain on medical services.

Note: personally, I know that drug treatment for mental conditions are very useful and they do have a place in treatment.

However, I want to stress the need for practitioners and everyone that drugs cannot solve certain causes of various conditions. Such as the impact of family, work and other factors can have on mental health.

Nonpharmacological Treatment:

Extremely interestingly, despite these treatments having a very negative perception in the media. There is a place for these treatments in modern practice.

I love these next few sections as they are shocking but very interesting.

Psychosurgery:

When I first read about this treatment option in my textbook, I was stunned because images of torture flooded my mind.

Also, it doesn't help that I use the idea of evil psychosurgery in my own sci-fi fantasy books.

Psychosurgery's Place in Modern Times:

Despite having a bad start with the majority of patients suffering from severe side effects. Like: impaired cognitive abilities.

Recently, psychosurgery has been refined a lot in both the procedures used as well as the assessment of the patient's sustainability. (Harley, Black, Stip and Taber, 2000)

Nowadays, psychosurgery is reserved as a last resort only to be used when all other treatment options no longer work.

Furthermore, instead of disconnecting or destroying entire lobes or brain regions. Surgeons only create lesions in certain areas of the brain.

I know that this sounds scary or concerning but a great example of psychosurgery is when the left and right hemispheres of the brain are disconnected from one another in patients suffering from severe epilepsy.

Meaning that these sufferers can live better lives.

Electroconvulsive Therapy:

This is another historically atrocious therapy, but modern versions look completely safe in comparison. As the modern treatment involves a brief 30-60 second shock that happens in 6-10 sessions over one to two weeks.

Moreover, patients are giving short-acting anaesthetic to make them temporarily unconscious so their seizure is restricted to only a few twitches. (Andreason and Black, 1996)

Interestingly, whilst this therapy was originally used to treat schizophrenia. It quickly becomes a preferred option to treat people with depression. (Andreasen and Black, 1996)

As a result, the therapy worked for 70%-90% of people who didn't respond to depression medication. (Andreasen and Black, 1996; Janicak et al, 1985)

On the other hand, this therapy is still controversial probably due to in many cases it can cause memory impairment. (Rami-Gonzalez et al, 2001)

Although, these cognitive impairments can be reduced if electricity is only applied to one side of the brain. (Sackeim et al, 2000)

Regardless of this fact, electroconvulsive therapy continues to be used only if medication has failed or if the patient is at a high risk of suicide. This has resulted in a clear consensus that this therapy is one of the effective treatment for depression.

If I had depression, I think that I would be

hoping that I responded to medication or psychotherapy because I would not want to experience this type of therapy.

Yet this does point out though that we must not dismiss any type of therapy unless it's unethical. As if this type of therapy was dismissed then all those people who suffered from depression would still be suffering.

Emerging Biomedical Treatment:

Below are some biomedical treatments that are at different stages of development and have the potential to help others:

- Vagal nerve stimulation- this is an emerging biomedical treatment option for depression. This works by using a small battery-powered implant that stimulus the vagal nerve.
- Deep brain stimulation- this biomedical treatment option is designed for people with depression or Obsessive Compulsive Disorder that involves stimulating very specific areas of the brain using implanted electrodes.
- Repetitive transcranial magnetic stimulation- emerging as a treatment for depression. This involves applying rapid sparks of magnetic stimulation to the brain from a coil that's held near the scalp.

Common Factors:

Finally, we've covered a lot of biological treatment options in this section and in the next few sections we will cover even more.

However, despite these treatments differing sometimes a lot from one another. all these therapies share the following:

- They are built upon relationships; like the therapeutic alliance; between the therapist and the patient.
- They give the sufferer hope of a better life.
- They develop new ways of thinking, behaving and feeling.

CHAPTER 15: PSYCHOLOGICAL TREATMENT

Now we're going to look at a very effective method of treatment, but it takes a long time. Its Cognitive Behavioural Therapy (CBT) the therapy is based on Beck's theory and it focuses on restructuring your mental processes and behavioural activation in order to change these automatic thoughts to be more positive.

Hollon et al (2005):

Three groups of patients with moderate to severe depression were compared.

They were people who had responded positively to CBT and had been withdrawn from medication for 12 months.

People who had responded and continued with medication.

People who had responded to medication and

continued to take a placebo.

Their relapse rates in 12 months were: CBT-31% Medication- 47% Placebo- 76%

In conclusion, CBT has a longer-lasting effect than medication.

Critically thinking:

The study shows the effectiveness of different treatments well and as it was over a long time period. We know that the effects of treatments over a long period of time.

However, this study fails to consider the other factors that could have caused a relapse. I believe that other factors like social factors could have caused the relapse instead of the treatment itself.

Fournier et al (2013):

Patients were assigned into one of three groups: CBT, medication and placebo.

Results were measured for mood, cognitive symptoms, vegetative symptoms and anxiety.

Results showed that CBT was more effective at targeting vegetative symptoms whereas medication was faster at reducing cognitive symptoms.

Summary:

CBT focuses on cognitive restructuring and behavioural activation.

Hollon et al (2005) shows that CBT has the longest-lasting effects of any treatment.

Fournier et al (2013) shows that CBT is best for targeting vegetative symptoms.

CHAPTER 16: ROLE OF CULTURE IN TREATMENT

Personally, I found this concept rather unusual at first. I suppose being from a western country I didn't see how culture could affect treatment.

However, when I started to think about it properly, I started to think that culture is vital for treatment.

As different cultures have different attitudes towards things like antidepressants and each culture has its own way of dealing with MDD.

For example: when I was taught this topic, we watched a video on how west Africa; if I remember correctly; treats depression and it was radically different to the west. As they made the whole village come together and support this person as they were covered in blood from a cow and then the village eats the cow as a BBQ.

I will admit that the memories are vague, but you get the essence of the idea and I quite like their idea about bringing the whole village together.

As I believe in the west that we are all too focused on ourselves and when people need us most, we are left to suffer, and so many people do fall through the cracks.

There are hundreds of case studies that support the idea of culture in treatment.

<u>Kinize et al (1987):</u>

Examined 41 depressed southeast Asian patients who were being treated with antidepressants in a US clinic.

Blood tests were run and it showed that 61% of patients were not taking the medication.

This is because of social stigma that is associated with taking antidepressants.

Cultural attitudes about authority caused patients to pretend to comply with the treatment as a way to not offend the doctors.

However, after a doctor-patient discussion about the benefits and problems of antidepressants. Compliance significantly improved.

Showing how an open discussion about cultural

beliefs can positively affect treatment.

Critically Thinking:

Overall, the study was effective at demonstrating how cultural attitudes can negatively affect treatment.

Although, to further support the findings and to add further creditability to the study. Follow up studies should be done using other cultures to see if the results are the same. Like: the Muslim population in New Zealand or the various African populations in the UK.

Griner and Smith (2006):

Meta-analysis of 76 studies with a qualitative section on their effectiveness was included.

Cultural adaptions ranged from familiarizing the therapist with the client's culture to training staff to be culturally sensitive.

Results showed that there were moderately strong benefits to cultural adaptions.

Treatment was more effective if the therapist spoke in the native tongue compared to English.

The benefit was 4 times stronger for same race client groups than mixed-race groups.

In conclusion, cultural adaptions for a specific

group of clients is more effective than making a general cultural adaptation.

Critically Thinking:

The study is effective as it uses a meta-analysis which can be used to increase the sample size of the studies by combining them, so the findings of the studies are more impactful.

However, this study could be open to publication bias; where only positive studies get published; as the study didn't state if it used published or a mixture of published and unpublished studies.

Summary:

Culture can impact treatment for many reasons.

Kinize et al (1987) shows that cultural attitudes can negatively impact treatment but having an open conversation can positively affect treatment.

Griner and Smith (2006) found that cultural adaptions for a specific group of clients are more effective than making a general cultural adaptation.

Bibliography:

Lee Parker (author), Darren Seath (author) Alexey Popov (author), *Oxford IB Diploma Programme: Psychology Course Companion,* 2nd edition, OUP Oxford, 2017

Alexey Popov, *IB Psychology Study Guide: Oxford IB Diploma Programme,* 2nd edition, OUP Oxford, 2018

https://www.medicalnewstoday.com/kc/serotonin-facts-232248

https://www.thinkib.net/psychology/page/22460/biological-approach-to-depression

Carr, A. (2012). Clinical Psychology: An Introduction. London: Routledge.

Davey G., Lake, N. and Whittington, A. (Eds). (2010). Clinical Psychology (2nd Edn). London: Routledge.

Almeida, O. P. et al. (2008). Low free testosterone concentration as a potentially treatable cause of depressive symptoms in older men. *Archives of General Psychiatry, 65,* 283-289.

Barton, D. A. et al. (2008). Elevated brain serotonin turnover in patients with depression. Effect of genotype and therapy. *Archives of General Psychiatry, 65,* 38-46.

Brunoni, A. R. et al. (2008). A systematic review and meta-analysis of clinical studies on major depression and BDNF levels: implications for the role of neuroplasticity in depression. *International Journal of Neuropsychopharmacology, 11,* 1169-1180.

Caparros-Gonzalez, R. A. et al. (2017). Hair cortisol levels, psychological stress, and psychopathological symptoms as predictors of postpartum depression. *PLOS One, 12,* e0182817.

Deuschle, M. et al. (1998). Borna disease virus proteins in cerebrospinal fluid of patients with recurrent depression and multiple sclerosis. *The Lancet, 352,* 1828-1829.

Giedke, H., & Schwarzler, F. (2002). Therapeutic use of sleep deprivation in depression. *Sleep Medicine Reviews, 6,* 361-377.

Harmer, C. J. et al. (2009). Why do antidepressants take so long to work? A cognitive neuropsychological model of antidepressant drug action. *The British Journal of Psychiatry, 195,* 102-108.

Kirsch I. et al. (2008). Initial Severity and Antidepressant Benefits: A Meta-Analysis of Data Submitted to the Food and Drug Administration. *PLoS Med 5,* e45.

Levinson, D. F. (2006). The genetics of depression: A review. *Biological Psychiatry, 60,* 84-92.

Rose, D. et al. (2003). Patients' perspectives on electroconvulsive therapy: systematic review. *British Medical Journal, 326,* 1363-1367.

UK ECT Review Group. (2003). Efficacy and safety of electroconvulsive therapy in depressive disorders: A systematic review and meta-analysis. *The Lancet, 361,* 799-808.

Callicott, J. H., et al. (2005). Variation in DISC1 affects hippocampal structure and function and increases risk for schizophrenia. *Proceedings of the National Academy of Sciences, 102,* 8627-8632.

Dimitrelis, K., & Shankar, R. (2016). Pharmacological treatment of schizophrenia – a review of progress. *Progress in Neurology and Psychiatry, 20,* 28-35.

Fatemi, S. H., & Folsom, T. D. The neurodevelopmental hypothesis of schizophrenia, revisited. *Schizophrenia Bulletin, 35,* 528-548.

Harrison, P. J. et al. (2003). Glutamate receptors and transporters in the hippocampus in schizophrenia. *Annals of the New York Academy of*

Sciences, 1003, 94-101.

Howes, O. D., & Kapur, S. (2009). The dopamine hypothesis of schizophrenia: Version II – The final common pathway. *Schizophrenia Bulletin, 35,* 549-562.

Ingraham, L. J. & Kety, S. S. (2000). Adoption studies of schizophrenia. *American Journal of Medical Genetics, 97,* 18-22.

Martinez, D. et al. (2007). Amphetamine-induced dopamine release: Markedly blunted in cocaine dependence and predictive of the choice to self-administer cocaine. *The American Journal of Psychiatry, 164,* 622-629.

Meltzer, H. Y., & Stahl, S. M. (1976). The dopamine hypothesis of schizophrenia: A review. *Schizophrenia Bulletin, 2,* 19-76.

Moghaddam, B. & Javitt, D. (2012). From revolution to evolution: The glutamate hypothesis of schizophrenia and its implication for treatment. *Neuropsychopharmacology, 37,* 4-15.

Murray, J. B. (2002). Phencyclidine (PCP): A dangerous drug but useful in schizophrenia research. *The Journal of Psychology, 163,* 319-327.

Murray, R. M., & Lewis, S. W. (1987). Is Schizophrenia a neurodevelopmental disorder? *British Medical Journal, 295,* 681-682.

Owen, M. J. et al. (2011). Neurodevelopmental hypothesis of schizophrenia. *The British Journal of Psychiatry, 198,* 173-175.

Saha, S. et al. (2005). A systematic review of the prevalence of schizophrenia. *PLOS Medicine, 2,* e141.

Sullivan, P. F. et al. (2003). Schizophrenia as a complex trait: Evidence from a meta-analysis of twin studies. *Archives of General Psychiatry, 60,* 1187-1192.

CONNOR WHITELEY

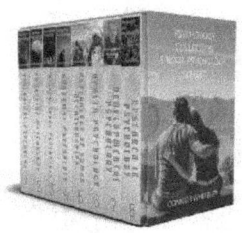
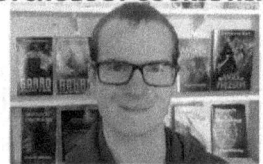

Thank you for reading.

I hoped you enjoyed it.

If you want a FREE book and keep up to date about new books and project. Then please sign up for my newsletter at www.connorwhiteley.net/

Have a great day.

CHECK OUT THE PSYCHOLOGY WORLD PODCAST FOR MORE PSYCHOLOGY INFORMATION!

AVAILABLE ON ALL MAJOR PODCAST APPS.

About the author:

Connor Whiteley is the author of over 20 books in the sci-fi fantasy, nonfiction psychology and books for writer's genre and he is a Human Branding Speaker and Consultant.

He is a passionate warhammer 40,000 reader, psychology student and author.

Who narrates his own audiobooks and he hosts The Psychology World Podcast.

All whilst studying Psychology at the University of Kent, England.

Also, he was a former Explorer Scout where he gave a speech to the Maltese President in August 2018 and he attended Prince Charles' 70th Birthday Party at Buckingham Palace in May 2018.

Plus, he is a self-confessed coffee lover!

Please follow me on:

Website: www.connorwhiteley.net

Twitter: @scifiwhiteley

Please leave on honest review as this helps with the discoverability of the book and I truly appreciate it.

Thank you for reading. I hope you've enjoyed.

All books in 'An Introductory Series':

BIOLOGICAL PSYCHOLOGY 3RD EDITION

COGNITIVE PSYCHOLOGY 2ND EDITION

SOCIAL PSYCHOLOGY- 3RD EDITION

ABNORMAL PSYCHOLOGY 3RD EDITION

PSYCHOLOGY OF RELATIONSHIPS- 3RD EDITION

DEVELOPMENTAL PSYCHOLOGY 3RD EDITION

HEALTH PSYCHOLOGY

RESEARCH IN PSYCHOLOGY

A GUIDE TO MENTAL HEALTH AND TREATMENT AROUND THE WORLD- A GLOBAL LOOK AT DEPRESSION

FORENSIC PSYCHOLOGY

CLINICAL PSYCHOLOGY

FORMULATION IN PSYCHOTHERAPY

63

Other books by Connor Whiteley:

THE ANGEL OF RETURN

THE ANGEL OF FREEDOM

GARRO: GALAXY'S END

GARRO: RISE OF THE ORDER

GARRO: END TIMES

GARRO: SHORT STORIES

GARRO: COLLECTION

GARRO: HERESY

GARRO: FAITHLESS

GARRO: DESTROYER OF WORLDS

GARRO: COLLECTIONS BOOK 4-6

GARRO: MISTRESS OF BLOOD

GARRO: BEACON OF HOPE

GARRO: END OF DAYS

WINTER'S COMING

WINTER'S HUNT

WINTER'S REVENGE

WINTER'S DISSENSION

Companion guides:

BIOLOGICAL PSYCHOLOGY 2ND EDITION WORKBOOK

COGNITIVE PSYCHOLOGY 2ND EDITION WORKBOOK

SOCIOCULTURAL PSYCHOLOGY 2ND EDITION WORKBOOK

ABNORMAL PSYCHOLOGY 2ND EDITION WORKBOOK

PSYCHOLOGY OF HUMAN RELATIONSHIPS 2ND EDITION WORKBOOK

HEALTH PSYCHOLOGY WORKBOOK

FORENSIC PSYCHOLOGY WORKBOOK

Audiobooks by Connor Whiteley:

BIOLOGICAL PSYCHOLOGY

COGNITIVE PSYCHOLOGY

SOCIOCULTURAL PSYCHOLOGY

ABNORMAL PSYCHOLOGY

PSYCHOLOGY OF HUMAN RELATIONSHIPS

HEALTH PSYCHOLOGY

DEVELOPMENTAL PSYCHOLOGY

RESEARCH IN PSYCHOLOGY

FORENSIC PSYCHOLOGY

GARRO: GALAXY'S END

GARRO: RISE OF THE ORDER

GARRO: SHORT STORIES

GARRO: END TIMES

GARRO: COLLECTION

GARRO: HERESY

GARRO: FAITHLESS

GARRO: DESTROYER OF WORLDS

GARRO: COLLECTION BOOKS 4-6

GARRO: COLLECTION BOOKS 1-6

Business books:

TIME MANAGEMENT: A GUIDE FOR STUDENTS AND WORKERS

LEADERSHIP: WHAT MAKES A GOOD LEADER? A GUIDE FOR STUDENTS AND WORKERS.

BUSINESS SKILLS: HOW TO SURVIVE THE BUSINESS WORLD? A GUIDE FOR STUDENTS, EMPLOYEES AND EMPLOYERS.

BUSINESS COLLECTION

GET YOUR FREE BOOK AT:
WWW.CONNORWHITELEY.NET

CPSIA information can be obtained
at www.ICGtesting.com
Printed in the USA
LVHW052030220321
682109LV00024B/1702